SACRAMENTO PUBLIC LIBRARY
3 3029 04820 6163

D1006667

COMPACT GUIDES TO FITNESS & HEALTH

YOUR GUIDE TO VITAMIN & MINERAL SUPPLEMENTS

CONTENT PROVIDED BY MAYO CLINIC HEALTH INFORMATION

MASON CREST PUBLISHERS
Philadelphia, Pennsylvania

Your Guide to Vitamin & Mineral Supplements provides reliable, practical, easy-to-understand information on substances for the healthy body. Much of the information comes directly from the experience of Mayo Clinic physicians, nurses, registered dietitians, health educators and other health care professionals. This book supplements the advice of your personal physician, whom you should consult for individual medical problems. MAYO, MAYO CLINIC, MAYO CLINIC HEALTH INFORMATION and the Mayo triple-shield logo are marks of Mayo Foundation for Medical Education and Research.

Hardcover Library Edition Published 2002
Mason Crest Publishers
370 Reed Road
Suite 302
Broomall, PA 19008-0914
(866) MCP-BOOK (toll free)

First Printing
1 2 3 4 5 6 7 8 9 10
Library of Congress Cataloging-in-Publication Data on file at the Library of Congress

ISBN 1-59084-262-6 (hc)
Printed in the United States of America

Contents

Vitamin and mineral basics 4
Whole foods are your best source. 6
Should you take supplements? 8
Vitamins and minerals:
How much do you need? 10
Daily Values for vitamins and minerals 11
Choosing and using supplements 12
Overviews of 15 vitamins and minerals 15
Vitamin A 15
Vitamin B-6 16
Vitamin B-12 17
Vitamin C 18
Vitamin D 19
Vitamin E 20
Folic acid/folate (Vitamin B-9) 22
Niacin (Vitamin B-3) 23
Beta carotene 24
Calcium 25
Iron 26
Magnesium 28
Potassium. 29
Selenium 30
Zinc 31
The final word: Food vs. supplements 32

Vitamin and mineral basics

Vitamins and minerals are substances your body needs in small amounts for normal growth, function and health. Together, vitamins and minerals are called micronutrients. Your body can't make most micronutrients, so you must get them from the foods you eat or, in some cases, from supplements.

Focus on vitamins

You need vitamins for normal body functions, mental alertness and resistance to infection. They enable your body to process proteins, carbohydrates and fats. Certain vitamins also help you produce blood cells, hormones, genetic material and chemicals in your nervous system. Unlike carbohydrates, proteins and fats, vitamins and minerals don't provide fuel (calories). However, they help your body release and use calories from food.

There are 14 vitamins, which fall into two categories:

- **Fat-soluble.** Vitamins A, D, E and K. They're stored in your body's fat. Some excess fat-soluble vitamins, such as Vitamins A and D, can accumulate in your body and reach toxic levels.
- **Water-soluble.** Vitamin C, choline, biotin and the seven B vitamins: thiamin (B-1), riboflavin (B-2), niacin (B-3), pantothenic acid (B-5), pyridoxine (B-6), folic acid/folate (B-9) and cobalamin (B-12). They're stored to a lesser extent than fat-soluble vitamins.

Focus on minerals

Your body also needs minerals. Major minerals (those needed in larger amounts) include calcium, phosphorus, magnesium, sodium, potassium and chloride. Calcium, phosphorus and magnesium are important in the development and health of bones and teeth. Sodium, potassium and chloride, known as electrolytes, are important in regulating the water and chemical balance in your body. In addition, your body needs smaller amounts of chromium, copper, fluoride, iodine, iron, manganese, molybdenum, selenium and zinc. These are all necessary for normal growth and health.

The right balance

Having the right balance of vitamins and minerals in your body is essential. Prolonged vitamin or mineral deficiencies can cause specific diseases or conditions, such as night blindness (vitamin A deficiency), pernicious anemia (vitamin B-12 deficiency) and anemia (iron deficiency). Too much of some vitamins and minerals can cause toxic reactions.

What's the difference between 'fortified' and 'enriched' foods?

These terms both indicate that nutrients have been added to a food. If a food or beverage is "fortified," it means that one or more nutrients have been added that weren't originally there. "Enriched" means that the nutrients lost during processing have been added back.

The Nutrition Facts listed on the label will tell you which nutrients have been added. They will also show what percentage of the Daily Value for each nutrient is met with one serving. (See "Daily Values for vitamins and minerals" on page 11.)

As you'll read on the next page, whole foods are the best source of nutrients for most people.

Whole foods are your best source

You can get your entire daily requirement of vitamin C by just popping a pill. You can get the same amount by eating a large orange. So which is better? In most cases, the orange — a whole food.

Benefits of whole foods

Whole foods — fruits, vegetables, grains, lean meats and dairy products — have three main benefits you can't find in a pill:

- **Whole foods are complex.** They contain a variety of the nutrients your body needs — not just one — giving you more "bang" for your nutrition "buck." An orange, for example, provides vitamin C but also beta carotene, calcium and other nutrients. A vitamin C supplement lacks these other nutrients. Similarly, a glass of milk provides you with protein, vitamin D, riboflavin, calcium, phosphorus and magnesium. If you take only calcium supplements and skip calcium-rich foods, such as dairy products, you may miss all the other nutrients you need for healthy bones.
- **Whole foods provide dietary fiber.** Fiber is important for digestion and it helps prevent certain diseases. Soluble fiber — found in certain beans and grains and in some fruits and vegetables — and insoluble fiber — found in whole grains and in some vegetables and fruits — may help prevent heart disease, diabetes and constipation.
- **Whole foods contain other substances that may be important for good health.** Fruits and vegetables, for example, contain naturally occurring food substances called phytochemicals, which may help protect you against cancer, heart disease, osteoporosis and diabetes. Although it's not yet known precisely what role phytochemicals play in nutrition, research shows many health benefits from eating more fruits, vegetables and grains.

If you depend on supplements rather than eating a variety of whole foods, you miss the potential benefits of phytochemicals.

Benefits of supplements uncertain

Only long-term, well-designed studies can sort out which nutrients in food are beneficial — and whether taking them in pill form provides the same benefit.

In fact, some nutrients may actually be harmful to your health when taken as a supplement. In one study, researchers found an increased risk of prostate cancer among men who drank alcohol and took beta carotene supplements. In an earlier study, they found that smokers who took beta carotene supplements had an increased risk of lung cancer. It's possible that alcohol and tobacco change the way your body absorbs and uses beta carotene. In addition, it's known that large amounts of beta carotene can alter blood levels of other similar natural food pigments called carotenoids, some of which may actually be more beneficial to you than beta carotene.

The bottom line

Concentrate on getting your nutrients from food, not supplements. Whole foods provide an ideal mix of nutrients, fiber and other food substances. It's likely that all of these work in combination to keep you healthy.

Should you take supplements?

The American Dietetic Association and other major medical organizations all agree that the best way to get the vitamins and minerals you need is through a nutritionally balanced diet. However, sometimes a supplement may be appropriate.

Even if you don't have a vitamin or mineral deficiency, a vitamin or mineral supplement may be appropriate for you if:

- **You're age 65 or older.** As you get older, health problems can contribute to a poor diet, making it difficult for you to get the vitamins and minerals you need. You may lose your appetite, as well as some of your ability to taste and smell. Depression or problems with dentures can also inhibit eating. If you eat alone, you also may not eat enough to get all the nutrients you need from food. In addition, as you get older, your body may not be able to absorb vitamins B-6, B-12 and D like it used to, making supplementation more necessary. There's also evidence that a multivitamin may improve your immune function and decrease your risk of some infections when you're older.

- **You're a postmenopausal woman.** For some women, it can be difficult to obtain the recommended amounts of calcium and vitamin D without supplementation. Both calcium and vitamin D supplements have been shown to protect against osteoporosis.

- **You don't eat well.** If you don't eat the recommended five servings a day of fruits and vegetables, taking a multivitamin supplement may be reasonable. However, your best course of action would be to adopt better eating habits.

- **You're on a very low-calorie diet.** If you eat less than 1,000 calories a day, you may benefit from a multivitamin-mineral supplement. However, remember: A very low-calorie diet limits the types and amounts of foods you eat and, in turn, the types and amounts of nutrients you receive. Very low-calorie diets should only be undertaken with guidance from your doctor.

• **You smoke.** Tobacco decreases absorption of many vitamins and minerals, including vitamin B-6, vitamin C, folic acid/folate and niacin. But supplements won't make up for the major health risks caused by smoking.

• **You drink alcohol excessively.** Long-term excessive alcohol consumption can impair digestion and absorption of thiamin, folic acid/folate and vitamins A, D and B-12. Altered metabolism also affects minerals such as zinc, selenium, magnesium and phosphorus. If you drink excessively, you also may substitute alcohol for food, resulting in a diet lacking in essential nutrients. Excessive drinking is defined as more than one drink on a daily basis for nonpregnant women or anyone age 65 or older, and more than two drinks a day for men.

• **You're pregnant or trying to become pregnant.** During this time, you need more of certain nutrients, especially calcium, folic acid and iron. Folic acid helps prevent neural tube defects, such as spina bifida, in your baby. Iron helps prevent fatigue by helping you make the red blood cells you need to deliver oxygen to your baby. Your doctor can recommend a supplement. It's important to start taking a supplement before becoming pregnant.

• **You eat a special diet.** If your diet has limited variety because of food allergies or intolerance to certain foods, you may benefit from a vitamin-mineral supplement. If you're a vegetarian who eliminates all animal products from your diet, you may need additional vitamin B-12. In addition, if you don't eat dairy products and don't get 15 minutes of sun each day on your skin, you may need to supplement your diet with calcium and vitamin D.

• **Your body can't absorb nutrients properly.** If you have a disease of your liver, gallbladder, intestine or pancreas, or you've had surgery on your digestive tract, you may not be able to digest and absorb nutrients properly. In such cases, your doctor may recommend that you take a vitamin or mineral supplement. A supplement may also be prescribed if you take antacids, antibiotics, laxatives or diuretics that interfere with nutrient absorption.

Vitamins and minerals: How much do you need?

You may be confused about how much of a specific vitamin or mineral you need. Here's how to figure out what you need:

- **Recommended Dietary Allowances (RDAs)** describe the average amount of each vitamin and mineral needed daily to meet the needs of nearly all healthy people. They're determined by the Food and Nutrition Board of the Institute of Medicine, part of the National Academy of Sciences. RDAs for some vitamins and minerals vary according to your sex, age and physical condition, for example, pregnancy.

- **Daily Values (DVs)** are used on food and supplement labels. (See "Daily Values for vitamins and minerals" on page 9.) They're set by the Food and Drug Administration (FDA), but the DVs are based on data that's much older than the data that's used to determine the RDAs. The FDA bases DVs on a 2,000-calorie-a-day diet. Of course, individual needs may vary.

  Many women and older adults may need only about 1,600 calories a day. Active women and most men need about 2,200 calories a day. Active men may need about 2,800 calories a day. If your calorie needs are greater or less than 2,000 a day, your DVs for various nutrients generally rise or fall accordingly.

- **Percent Daily Value (%DV)** tells you what percentage of the DV one serving of a food or supplement supplies. For example, if the label on your multivitamin bottle says that your multivitamin provides 30 percent of the DV for vitamin E, you'll need another 70 percent to meet the recommended goal.

Daily Values for vitamins and minerals

If you decide to use a supplement, experts recommend choosing one that doesn't exceed 100 percent of the Daily Value for each vitamin and mineral, unless your doctor advises otherwise. Daily Values are listed on supplement labels. They're based on a daily intake of 2,000 calories and meet or exceed recommended vitamin and mineral needs for most people. (See page 8 for a definition of Daily Value.)

VITAMIN	100% DAILY VALUE
Vitamin A*	5,000 international units (IU)*
Vitamin C	60 milligrams (mg)
Vitamin D	400 IU
Vitamin E	20 IU natural source or 30 IU synthetic source
Vitamin K	80 micrograms (mcg)
Thiamin (vitamin B-1)	1.5 mg
Riboflavin (vitamin B-2)	1.7 mg
Niacin (vitamin B-3)	20 mg
Pantothenic acid (vitamin B-5)	10 mg
Pyridoxine (vitamin B-6)	2 mg
Folic acid/folate (vitamin B-9)	0.4 mg or 400 mcg
Cobalamin (vitamin B-12)	6 mcg
Biotin	0.3 mg or 300 mcg

MINERAL	100% DAILY VALUE
Calcium	1,000 mg or 1 gram (g)
Chloride	3,400 mg
Chromium	120 mcg
Copper	2 mg
Iodine	150 mcg
Iron**	18 mg**
Magnesium	400 mg
Manganese	2 mg
Molybdenum	75 mcg
Phosphorus	1,000 mg
Potassium	3,500 mg
Selenium	70 mcg
Zinc	15 mg

*New Recommended Dietary Allowances (RDAs) are lower: 3,000 IU a day for men and 2,330 IU a day for most women. (See the RDA chart for vitamin A on page 13.)

**For men and postmenopausal women, it's probably wise to use a pill with little (8 mg a day or less) or no iron.

Choosing and using supplements

Supplements are not substitutes. They can't replace the hundreds of nutrients in whole foods you need for a nutritionally balanced diet. However, if you do decide to take a vitamin or mineral supplement, here are some factors to consider:

- **Avoid supplements that provide "megadoses."** In general, choose a multivitamin-mineral supplement that provides about 100% DV of all the vitamins and minerals instead of one that supplies, for example, 500% DV of one vitamin and only 20% DV of another. The exception to this is calcium. You may notice that

Multivitamins: Do you need one?

Because diets of older people are often short in more than one vitamin and mineral, a multivitamin-mineral pill taken once a day may make more sense than single-nutrient pills. Look for a supplement that contains a wide variety of vitamins and minerals in the appropriate amounts, usually 100 percent of the Daily Value (DV).

Check the contents to make sure you're not getting too much of any nutrient, which can be harmful. In most cases, if the tablet doesn't exceed 100 percent of the DV, it's considered safe. Talk with your doctor or pharmacist if you have questions.

Here are a few things to consider when choosing a multivitamin-mineral pill:

- **Iron.** Although supplemental iron is advised during pregnancy and for iron deficiency anemia, some studies suggest that excess iron can raise the risk of heart disease and colon cancer for women beyond menopause and for men. For these people, it's probably wise to use a pill with little or no iron (8 mg or less).

calcium-containing supplements don't provide 100% DV. If they did, the tablets would be too large to swallow. Most cases of nutrient toxicity stem from high-dose supplements.

• **Look for USP on the label.** This ensures that the supplement meets the standards for strength, purity, disintegration and dissolution established by the testing organization, U.S. Pharmacopeia (USP).

• **Beware of gimmicks.** Synthetic vitamins are the same as so-called "natural" vitamins. Don't give in to the temptation of added herbs, enzymes or amino acids — they add nothing but cost.

• **Vitamin B-6 (pyridoxine).** Adequate levels of this vitamin may help lower blood homocysteine, a risk factor for heart attack, and improve your immune system function. Older people have trouble absorbing it, so a multivitamin that contains about 2 mg is often a good idea. Avoid excessive doses. Too much vitamin B-6 can result in nerve damage to the arms and legs, which is usually reversible when supplementation is stopped.

• **Vitamin B-12 (cobalamin).** Adequate levels of this vitamin may reduce your risk of anemia, cardiovascular disease and stroke. Older people often don't absorb this vitamin well. A multivitamin with at least 2 micrograms (mcg) may help.

• **Vitamin D.** This vitamin helps the body absorb calcium and is essential in maintaining proper bone strength and bone density. Because many older people don't get regular exposure to sunlight and have trouble absorbing this vitamin, taking a multivitamin with 400 international units (IU) will probably help improve bone health.

• **Vitamin E.** Studies on the benefits of vitamin E show mixed results. If you're taking blood-thinning medications or have any of the conditions listed under "Cautions" on page 21, talk with your doctor before taking a supplement containing vitamin E.

• **Look for expiration dates.** Supplements can lose potency over time, especially in hot and humid climates. If a supplement doesn't have an expiration date, don't buy it.

• **Store all vitamin and mineral supplements out of the sight and reach of children.** Put them in a locked cabinet or other secured location. Don't leave them sitting out on the counter or rely on child-resistant packaging. Be especially careful with any supplements containing iron. Iron overdose is a leading cause of poisoning deaths among children.

• **Store supplements in a dry, cool place.** Avoid hot, humid storage locations, such as the bathroom.

• **Explore your options.** If you have difficulty swallowing, ask your doctor whether a chewable or liquid form of the vitamin and mineral supplements might be right for you.

• **Play it safe.** Before taking anything other than a standard multivitamin-mineral supplement of 100% DV or less, check with your doctor, pharmacist or a registered dietitian. This is especially important if you have a health problem or are taking medication. High doses of niacin, for example, can result in liver problems. In addition, supplements may interfere with medications. Vitamins E and K, for example, aren't recommended if you're taking blood-thinning medications (anticoagulants) because they can complicate the proper control of blood thinning. If you're already taking an individual vitamin or mineral supplement and haven't told your doctor, discuss it at your next checkup.

Overviews of 15 vitamins and minerals

Here's what you need to know about 15 popular vitamins and minerals — how much you need, what they do for your body, good food sources, cautions and side effects.

Vitamin A

Recommended Dietary Allowance (RDA) for Adults

Life stage	Men	Women	Pregnant	Breast-feeding
Age 19 or older	3,000 IU or 900 mcg/day	2,330 IU or 700 mcg/day		
Other			2,565 IU or 770 mcg/day	4,335 IU or 1,300 mcg/day

IU = international units (labels usually list Vitamin A in IU); mcg = micrograms

Maximum daily intake (from all sources) unlikely to pose risk of side effects for adults: 10,000 IU or 3,000 mcg/day (Some experts recommend a maximum of 5,000 IU or 1,500 mcg/day for pregnant women.)

Food sources include: Animal sources such as whole milk, fat-free milk fortified with vitamin A, whole eggs, liver, beef and chicken. Plant sources of beta carotene, which converts into vitamin A, include dark green leafy vegetables and orange and yellow fruits, such as carrots, sweet potatoes, spinach, broccoli, cantaloupe, mangos, apricots, as well as vegetable soup and tomato juice.

What it does: Vitamin A is a fat-soluble vitamin that plays a role in healthy vision, bone growth and reproduction. It also helps to regulate your immune system, which is important to prevent and fight infections. Inadequate amounts of vitamin A can cause vision impairment, especially at night.

What the research says: Your body can convert plant sources of beta carotene into vitamin A, but animal sources of vitamin A are better absorbed. So vegetarians who rely on fruits and vegetables rich in beta carotene to meet their daily vitamin A requirement need to eat at least five daily servings of such foods. Two national surveys in the 1990s indicated that some Americans don't eat enough foods rich in vitamin A. However, vitamin A deficiency is rare in the United States — it's more often associated with malnutrition, a leading problem in developing countries. But people with certain diseases who have trouble absorbing vitamin A may have supplements recommended by their doctors. Surveys suggest a link between diets that are rich in vitamin A and beta carotene from food — not supplements — and a lower risk of some types of cancer.

Cautions: Too much vitamin A stored in the body may increase the risks of birth defects and liver abnormalities and reduce bone mineral density, which could result in osteoporosis. If you're pregnant or breast-feeding, don't take vitamin A in doses greater than the RDA for pregnant or breast-feeding women.

Side effects: Signs and symptoms of vitamin A toxicity include nausea and vomiting, headache, dizziness, blurred vision and problems with muscular coordination. Most cases of vitamin A toxicity result from an excess intake of vitamin A supplements. Plant sources of beta carotene, which converts to vitamin A, are generally considered safe. A high intake of beta carotene from plant sources can turn the skin an orange color, but this is not considered a health concern. However, the safety of beta carotene *supplements* is questionable. (See "Beta carotene" on page 24.)

Vitamin B-6 (Pyridoxine)

Recommended Dietary Allowance (RDA) for Adults

Life stage	Men	Women	Pregnant	Breast-feeding
Ages 19 to 50	1.3 mg/day	1.3 mg/day		
Age 51 or older	1.7 mg/day	1.5 mg/day		
Other			1.9 mg/day	2.0 mg/day

mg = milligrams

Maximum daily intake (from all sources) unlikely to pose risk of side effects for adults: 100 mg/day

Food sources include: Poultry, fish, pork, eggs, soybeans, oats, whole-grain products, nuts, seeds and bananas. One medium banana contains 0.7 mg of vitamin B-6.

What it does: Vitamin B-6 is a water-soluble vitamin that is essential for protein metabolism, energy production and normal brain function.

What the research says: Vitamin B-6 has been shown to work together with vitamin B-12 and folic acid/folate to reduce blood levels of homocysteine, an amino acid that builds and maintains tissues. Elevated homocysteine levels can increase your risk of heart attack, stroke or loss of circulation in your hands and feet. Many people tout vitamin B-6 as a remedy for premenstrual syndrome (PMS). However, studies have shown conflicting results. Large doses taken to treat carpal tunnel or premenstrual syndromes have been associated with neurological problems and skin lesions.

Cautions: See your doctor before taking vitamin B-6 if you have intestinal problems, liver disease, an overactive thyroid, sickle cell disease or if you've been under severe stress as a result of illness, burns, an accident or recent surgery. If you're pregnant or breast-feeding, don't take vitamin B-6 in doses greater than the RDA for pregnant or breast-feeding women.

Side effects: High daily doses of vitamin B-6, especially over 250 mg/day, may cause nerve damage.

Vitamin B-12 (Cobalamin)

Recommended Dietary Allowance (RDA) for Adults

Life stage	Men	Women	Pregnant	Breast-feeding
Age 19 or older	2.4 mcg/day	2.4 mcg/day		
Other			2.6 mcg/day	2.8 mcg/day

mcg = micrograms

Maximum daily intake (from all sources) unlikely to pose risk of side effects for adults: There is no known toxicity in humans from vitamin B-12.

Food sources include: Meat, fish, shellfish, poultry, eggs and dairy products. A portion (3 ounces) of lean sirloin contains 2.2 mcg of vitamin B-12. Fortified breakfast cereals may also contain vitamin B-12 — check the label.

What it does: Vitamin B-12 is a water-soluble vitamin that has essential roles in red blood cell formation, cell metabolism and nerve function.

What the research says: Vitamin B-12 supplements containing 100% of the Daily Value (6 mcg a day) help prevent deficiency in vegetarians who eliminate all animal foods from their diets. (Plant foods don't contain vitamin B-12.) Injections of vitamin B-12 prevent and treat deficiency in people whose digestive tracts can't absorb vitamin B-12, whether because of surgery, bowel disease or a hereditary problem. Up to 15 percent of people over age 60 may have vitamin B-12 deficiency.

Cautions: See your doctor before taking vitamin B-12 if you have anemia with no known cause. If you're pregnant or breast-feeding, don't take vitamin B-12 in doses greater than the RDA for pregnant or breast-feeding women.

Side effects: The Institute of Medicine reports that no adverse effects have been linked with excess vitamin B-12 intake from food and supplements in healthy people.

Additional information: If you're over age 50, your body is less able to absorb vitamin B-12 from animal foods as you age. You may need to get your vitamin B-12 through supplements or fortified foods. If you have vitamin B-12 deficiency (pernicious anemia) or have had a portion of your gastrointestinal tract surgically removed, your body can't absorb enough of an oral vitamin. In such cases, your doctor will likely recommend vitamin B-12 through injections.

Vitamin C (Ascorbic Acid)

Recommended Dietary Allowance (RDA) for Adults

Life stage	Men	Women	Pregnant	Breast-feeding
Age 19 or older	90 mg/day	75 mg/day		
Adult smokers	125 mg/day	110 mg/day		
Other			85 mg/day	120 mg/day

mg = milligrams

Maximum daily intake (from all sources) unlikely to pose risk of side effects for adults: 2,000 mg/day

Food sources include: Citrus juices and fruits, berries, tomatoes, potatoes, green and red peppers, broccoli and spinach. One cup (8 ounces) reconstituted orange juice contains about 100 mg of vitamin C.

What it does: Vitamin C is a water-soluble vitamin that maintains skin integrity, helps heal wounds and is important in immune functions. It also has antioxidant properties, helping to prevent cell damage by neutralizing "free radicals" — molecules believed to be associated with aging and certain diseases.

What the research says: Studies have shown that people who eat foods high in vitamin C have lower rates of cancer and heart disease, though it's unclear whether taking vitamin C supplements produces similar benefits. A 2001 study indicates that supplementation with vitamin C, certain other antioxidants and zinc may slow the progression of age-related macular degeneration, but a doctor's supervision is important to determine proper doses. The Institute of Medicine states that there are no established benefits for consuming vitamin C in doses higher than the RDA. Other research has suggested that 200 mg/day is the optimal dose.

Cautions: See your doctor before taking vitamin C if you have gout, kidney stones, sickle cell anemia or iron storage disease. If you're pregnant or breast-feeding, don't take vitamin C in doses greater than the RDA for pregnant or breast-feeding women.

Side effects: Taking excessive amounts of vitamin C (over 2,000 mg/day) may cause mild diarrhea. It may also interfere with stool tests for blood and other laboratory tests.

Vitamin D (Calciferol)

Adequate Intake (AI) for Adults*

Life stage	Men and women	Pregnant or breast-feeding
Ages 19 to 50	200 IU or 5 mcg/day	
Ages 51 to 70	400 IU or 10 mcg/day	
Age 71 or older	600 IU or 15 mcg/day	
Other		200 IU or 5 mcg/day

IU = international units (labels usually list vitamin D in IU); mcg = micrograms
*AI levels are used because the Recommended Dietary Allowance (RDA) has not been established.

Maximum daily intake (from all sources) unlikely to pose risk of side effects for adults: 2,000 IU or 50 mcg/day

Food sources include: Vitamin D-fortified milk, vitamin D-fortified cereal, liver, egg yolks, fish and fish liver oils. One cup (8 ounces) of vitamin D-fortified milk contains 100 IU.

What it does: Vitamin D is necessary for effective absorption of dietary calcium. It also helps deposit calcium in your bones and teeth.

What the research says: Your body gets vitamin D from dietary sources, but it can also generate its own when sunlight converts a chemical in your skin into a usable form of the vitamin. However, some people don't get enough vitamin D due to lack of exposure to sunlight, less efficient conversion of the vitamin in their skin or reduced liver or kidney function. If you don't drink milk, have dark skin, are at risk of osteoporosis, live in a cloudy environment or rarely go outside, you may want to consider taking a vitamin D supplement to meet your daily requirement. Studies show that people who supplement their diets with a combination of vitamin D and calcium slow bone loss and reduce the number of fractures.

Cautions: See your doctor before taking vitamin D if you have epilepsy, heart or blood vessel disease, chronic diarrhea, disease of the kidney, liver or pancreas, intestinal problems, sarcoidosis (an immune system disorder) or if you're planning to become pregnant. If you're pregnant or breast-feeding, don't take vitamin D in doses greater than the RDA for pregnant or breast-feeding women.

Side effects: Prolonged intake of vitamin D above 2,000 IU/day poses the risk of toxic effects. Side effects can include nausea, headache, excessive urination, high blood pressure, deposits of calcium in soft tissues, kidney damage and other problems.

Vitamin E (Tocopherol)

Recommended Dietary Allowance (RDA) for Adults

Life stage	Men and women	Pregnant	Breast-feeding
Age 19 or older	15 mg/day or 22 IU natural source or 33 IU synthetic source*		
Other		15 mg/day or 22 IU natural source or 33 IU synthetic source*	19 mg/day or 28 IU natural source or 42 IU synthetic source*

IU = international units (labels usually list vitamin E in IU); mg = milligrams
*The natural source is called d-alpha-tocopherol on the supplement label. The synthetic source is called dl-alpha-tocopherol on the label.

Maximum daily intake (from supplements and fortified foods) unlikely to pose risk of side effects for adults: 1,500 IU natural source or 1,100 IU synthetic source (1,000 mg)/day

Food sources include: Vegetable oils, wheat germ, whole-grain products, avocados and nuts. Two tablespoons of peanut butter contain 3 mg of vitamin E.

What it does: Vitamin E is a fat-soluble vitamin that protects red blood cells and is important in reproduction. It also has antioxidant properties, helping to prevent cell damage by neutralizing "free radicals" — molecules believed to be associated with aging and certain diseases.

What the research says: Vitamin E is a potent antioxidant that attaches directly to low-density lipoprotein (LDL) cholesterol (the "bad" cholesterol) in your blood and helps prevent damage from free radicals. Some studies show that it might prevent or slow progression of plaques forming within your artery walls (atherosclerosis) if you have heart disease or diabetes. However, other recent studies show no benefit from vitamin E supplements in high-risk heart patients. Some studies suggest that vitamin E may slow the progression of Parkinson's disease and Alzheimer's disease, enhance immunity in older adults, and help prevent prostate cancer, but more research is needed. A 2001 study indicates that supplementation with vitamin E, certain other antioxidants and zinc may slow the progression of age-related macular degeneration, but a doctor's supervision is important to determine proper doses to lower the risk of side effects.

Although some studies on the benefits of vitamin E supplements appear promising, it's important to remember two things. First, when it comes to preventing heart disease, any benefits from vitamin E supplements are much less than you get from exercising, eating a healthy diet and managing other risk factors, such as high blood pressure and high cholesterol. Second, there isn't enough evidence yet to recommend vitamin E supplements for the general population.

Cautions: Check with your doctor first before taking vitamin E if you're taking blood-thinning (anticoagulant) medications. Vitamin E can complicate the proper control of blood thinning. See your doctor before taking vitamin E if you have iron deficiency anemia, bleeding or clotting problems, cystic fibrosis, intestinal problems or liver disease. If you're pregnant or breast-feeding, don't take vitamin E in doses greater than the RDA for pregnant or breast-feeding women.

Side effects: In rare cases, people who take vitamin E may develop dizziness, fatigue, headache, weakness, abdominal pain, diarrhea, flu-like symptoms, nausea or blurred vision. At high doses (above 1,500 IU natural or 1,100 IU synthetic source/day), vitamin E can cause side effects that can include bleeding — especially for people on blood-thinning medications — and gastrointestinal complaints. However, in general, vitamin E is very well tolerated by most people.

Folic acid/folate (Vitamin B-9)

Recommended Dietary Allowance (RDA) for Adults

Life stage	Men and women	Pregnant	Breast-feeding
Age 19 or older	400 mcg/day		
Other		600 mcg/day	500 mcg/day

mcg = micrograms

Maximum daily intake (from supplements and fortified foods) unlikely to pose risk of side effects for adults: 1,000 mcg/day

Food sources include: Citrus juices and fruits, beans, nuts, seeds, liver, dark green leafy vegetables and fortified grain products (bread, pasta, breakfast cereals, rice). Half a cup (4 ounces) of cooked spinach contains 130 mcg of folate.

What it does: Folate, also called vitamin B-9, occurs naturally in certain foods (see above). Folic acid is the synthetic form of folate. Folic acid is found in supplements and in fortified breads and cereals. This water-soluble vitamin is important in red blood cell formation, protein metabolism, growth and cell division. It's also very important in pregnancy for the developing fetus.

What the research says: Folic acid has been shown to work together with vitamin B-6 and vitamin B-12 to reduce blood levels of homocysteine, an amino acid that builds and maintains tissues. Elevated homocysteine levels can increase your risk of heart attack, stroke or loss of circulation in your hands and feet. Folic acid also helps prevent neural tube defects, such as spina bifida, in developing fetuses — if taken before and during pregnancy. If you don't get adequate folate in your diet, consider taking a folic acid supplement.

Cautions: See your doctor before taking folic acid if you have anemia. Intake of folic acid from supplements and fortified foods shouldn't exceed 1,000 mcg a day to prevent folic acid from covering up the symptoms of a vitamin B-12 deficiency. Follow your doctor's recommendation if you're taking folic acid for any medical reasons.

Side effects: People who take folic acid may develop bright yellow urine, fever, shortness of breath, a skin rash or, very rarely, diarrhea. Doses over 1,500 mcg/day can cause nausea, appetite loss, flatulence and abdominal distention.

Niacin (Vitamin B-3)

Recommended Dietary Allowance (RDA) for Adults

Life stage	Men	Women	Pregnant	Breast-feeding
Age 19 or older	16 mg/day	14 mg/day		
Other			18 mg/day	17 mg/day

mg = milligrams

Maximum daily intake (from supplements and fortified foods) unlikely to pose risk of side effects for adults: 35 mg/day

Food sources include: Lean meats, poultry, fish, organ meats, brewer's yeast, peanuts and peanut butter. A portion (3 ounces) of lean sirloin contains 3 mg of niacin.

What it does: Niacin is a water-soluble B vitamin important in energy metabolism.

What the research says: Niacin can reduce lipids in your blood, including lowering low-density lipoprotein (LDL) cholesterol (the "bad" cholesterol) and triglycerides, and raising high-density lipoprotein (HDL) cholesterol (the "good" cholesterol). Studies show that niacin can also slow the progression of atherosclerosis when used with other cholesterol-lowering drugs, diet and exercise. However, in the doses typically needed for these effects (usually greater than 1,000 mg/day), niacin is being used as a medication, not as a vitamin. So take increased doses only with your doctor's advice.

Cautions: Don't take niacin if you have impaired liver function or an active peptic ulcer. See your doctor before taking niacin if you have diabetes, gout, gallbladder or liver disease, arterial bleeding or glaucoma. If you're pregnant or breast-feeding, don't take niacin in doses greater than the RDA for pregnant or breast-feeding women.

Side effects: At doses of higher than 2,000 mg/day, niacin has potentially serious side effects that can include liver damage, high blood sugar and irregular heartbeats. As little as 50 mg/day can cause flushing, itching, headaches, cramps and nausea.

Beta carotene

Recommended Dietary Allowance (RDA): None established*

Maximum daily intake unlikely to pose risk of side effects for adults: None established*

*The Food and Nutrition Board of the Institute of Medicine states that beta carotene *supplements* are not advisable for the general population, although doctors may recommend this supplement for people who have vitamin A deficiency.

Food sources include: Carrots, cantaloupe, pumpkin, sweet potatoes and tomatoes.

What it does: Beta carotene is one of more than 600 carotenoid compounds found in animals, plants and microorganisms. Your body converts beta carotene into vitamin A, a fat-soluble vitamin essential for vision, growth, cell division, reproduction and immunity.

What the research says: Some studies indicate that diets high in beta carotene and other carotenoids *obtained from food* are associated with a lower risk of chronic diseases such as heart disease and some cancers. However, this effect may be due to other substances found in carotenoid-rich foods, not only beta carotene. Several well-designed studies have found that supplements of beta carotene offer no protection against heart disease. Three large clinical trials found that beta carotene supplements did not protect against cancer. Two studies found an increased risk of lung cancer among smokers who took beta carotene supplements, and one found an increased risk of prostate cancer among men who took beta carotene supplements and also drank alcohol. A large Finnish study found that daily supplements of beta carotene had no effect on the prevalence of cataracts. A recent study indicates that a small amount of beta carotene taken with certain other antioxidants and zinc may slow the progression of age-related macular degeneration, but a doctor's supervision is important to determine proper doses to lower the risk of side effects.

Cautions: Avoid taking beta carotene supplements because of the risks noted above, unless your doctor advises otherwise. If you smoke, taking beta carotene supplements may increase your risk of lung cancer. If you're seeking the potential benefits of beta carotene, eat more red and yellow vegetables. (See food sources above.)

Side effects: People who take beta carotene may develop an orange color to their skin, which is reversible when beta carotene is discontinued.

Calcium

Recommended Dietary Allowance (RDA) for Adults

Life stage	Men and women	Pregnant or breast-feeding
Ages 19 to 50	1,000 mg/day	
Age 51 or older	1,200 mg/day	
Other		1,000 mg/day

mg = milligrams

Maximum daily intake (from all sources) unlikely to pose risk of side effects for adults: 2,500 mg/day

Food sources include: Milk and milk products, fish with bones that are eaten, calcium-fortified tofu, calcium-fortified orange juice and broccoli. One cup (8 ounces) of milk contains 300 mg of calcium.

What it does: Calcium is a mineral important for strong teeth and bones and for muscle and nerve function.

What the research says: Studies suggest that calcium supplements, if taken regularly, help prevent osteoporosis by reducing bone loss. The question is how much calcium you need to achieve this. Although the RDA for calcium is 1,200 mg a day for adults age 51 or older, some experts believe that some people may need more than that. They recommend calcium in doses of 1,500 mg/day for men over age 65 and postmenopausal women not taking estrogen replacement therapy. If you don't get enough calcium in your diet, consider taking a supplement. You may even experience some side benefits. A 1998 study found that women who took 1,200 mg/day of chewable calcium carbonate reduced the physical and psychological symptoms of premenstrual syndrome (PMS) by 20 percent more than those taking a placebo. In addition, a 14-year study of 86,000 women found that those who had a relatively high intake of calcium, whether through diet or use of supplements, had a reduced risk of stroke.

Cautions: Don't take calcium if you have sarcoidosis (an immune system disorder) or a high blood-calcium level. See your doctor before taking calcium if you have kidney disease, chronic constipation, colitis, diarrhea, stomach or intestinal bleeding, irregular heartbeat or heart problems. If you're pregnant or breast-feeding, don't take calcium in doses greater than the RDA for pregnant or breast-feeding women. However, if you don't get enough calcium in your diet, ask your doctor whether calcium supplements are right for you.

Side effects: People who take calcium supplements may experience constipation and headache. Serious side effects include confusion, muscle or bone pain, nausea, vomiting, and slow or irregular heartbeat.

Additional information: Chewable calcium tablets and calcium powders and solutions may be more easily absorbed than hard, compressed calcium tablets. Avoid calcium supplements made from bone meal, dolomite or oyster shell, often advertised as "natural." These may contain toxic substances, such as lead, mercury and arsenic. Limit single doses to no more than 500 mg elemental (available) calcium. If you take an iron supplement, don't take it at the same time as your calcium supplement. Calcium can interfere with the absorption of iron.

Iron

Recommended Dietary Allowance (RDA) for Adults

Life stage	Men	Women	Pregnant	Breast-feeding
Ages 19 to 50	8 mg/day	18 mg/day*		
Age 51 or older	8 mg/day	8 mg/day**		
Other			27 mg/day	9 mg/day**

mg = milligrams
*Women who are menstruating
**Women who are not menstruating

Maximum daily intake (from all sources) unlikely to pose risk of side effects for adults: 45 mg/day

Food sources: There are two types of dietary iron.

- Heme iron, which the body usually absorbs well, is found in meat, seafood and poultry. A portion (3 ounces) of beef, pork, lamb or veal contains 2 to 3 mg of iron.
- Nonheme iron, which isn't absorbed as well as heme iron, is found in iron-fortified cereals, whole grains, beans (for example, kidney, pinto, lima and navy beans), peas, and dark leafy green veg-

etables (for example, spinach). Because absorption of nonheme iron is lower, vegetarians who don't consume any animal products may require higher amounts of dietary iron. The body better absorbs nonheme iron from plant foods when they're consumed along with a reliable source of vitamin C, such as citrus fruits.

What it does: Iron is a mineral that is an essential constituent of blood and muscle and important for the transport of oxygen.

What the research says: When there is not enough iron in your diet, too few red blood cells are made to adequately carry oxygen. This condition is called iron deficiency anemia and can affect women of childbearing age and people with conditions that cause internal bleeding, such as ulcers or intestinal diseases. But for healthy men and postmenopausal women, iron deficiency is rare. If you want to make sure you're getting enough iron, your best bet is to eat a nutritionally balanced diet containing iron-rich foods.

Cautions: Don't take iron if you have acute hepatitis, hemosiderosis or hemochromatosis (conditions involving excess iron in the body), hemolytic anemia or if you've had repeated blood transfusions. See your doctor before taking iron if you've had peptic ulcer disease, enteritis, colitis, pancreatitis or hepatitis. Also see your doctor if you have kidney disease, intestinal disease, consume excessive alcohol or if you plan to become pregnant. If you're pregnant or breast-feeding, ask your doctor whether supplements with iron are right for you. And if you're over age 55 and have a family history of heart disease, consult your doctor before taking iron.

Side effects: Iron supplements can cause side effects in some people, such as nausea, vomiting, constipation, diarrhea, dark-colored stools and abdominal pain. Taking the supplement in divided doses and with food may help avoid or limit these signs and symptoms. Liquid iron can cause tooth stain. Because overdose of iron medication can be toxic to young children, keep iron supplements tightly capped and out of reach.

Magnesium

Recommended Dietary Allowance (RDA) for Adults

Life stage	Men	Women	Pregnant	Breast-feeding
Ages 19 to 30	400 mg/day	310 mg/day	350 mg/day	310 mg/day
Age 31 or older	420 mg/day	320 mg/day	360 mg/day	320 mg/day

mg = milligrams

Maximum daily intake (from supplements only) unlikely to pose risk of side effects for adults: 350 mg/day

Food sources include: Nuts, legumes, whole grains and dark green vegetables. Half a cup (4 ounces) of kidney beans contains 40 mg of magnesium.

What it does: Magnesium is a mineral necessary in many enzyme processes. It helps your nerves and muscles function properly.

What the research says: A 1998 study found that magnesium supplements (200 mg/day) reduced fluid retention, breast tenderness and bloating by 40 percent among women with premenstrual syndrome (PMS). Infusions of magnesium may also relieve headache pain in some people who suffer from migraines. Ask your doctor if this treatment might be right for you. Though some scientists have proposed that magnesium supplements may help keep bones strong, there's currently not enough medical evidence to support this view.

Cautions: Don't take magnesium supplements if you're pregnant or breast-feeding, or if you have kidney failure or heart block (unless you have a pacemaker) or have had an ileostomy. See your doctor before taking magnesium if you have stomach or intestinal bleeding, symptoms of appendicitis or chronic constipation, colitis or diarrhea.

Side effects: People who take magnesium supplements may experience abdominal cramps, appetite loss, diarrhea, irregular heartbeat, mood changes, fatigue, nausea, vomiting or pain when urinating. When taken with food, magnesium supplements are less likely to cause diarrhea, nausea and abdominal cramps. If you're over age 55 and take magnesium supplements, you're at increased risk of side effects.

Additional information: Certain antacids may provide significant magnesium — check the label.

Potassium

Recommended Dietary Allowance (RDA): None established*

*RDAs have not been established and potassium deficiency is rare, except for certain circumstances. See "What the research says" below.

Maximum daily intake (from all sources) unlikely to pose risk of side effects for adults: None established. The Daily Value is 3,500 milligrams (mg)/day, which most people can get from food sources. (See "Daily Values" for vitamins and minerals on page 9.)

Food sources include: Citrus fruits (such as oranges), apples, bananas, apricots, cantaloupe, potatoes (especially with skin), tomatoes, spinach, mushrooms, beans and peas, among other foods.

What it does: Potassium is one of the minerals responsible for maintaining the electrical stability of the cells of your heart and nervous system. It's also called an electrolyte. Potassium is important for cell and muscle growth, and it plays a major role in maintaining normal fluid balance.

What the research says: Most people get all the potassium they need from eating a balanced diet. Potassium deficiency is rare, but your doctor may recommend potassium supplements if you don't get enough because of a medical condition or certain medications. For example, some high blood pressure medications (diuretics) increase urination, which could lead to potassium deficiency. Some studies indicate that low potassium may contribute to high blood pressure and that increasing potassium intake through diet may prevent or help treat hypertension. Some studies indicate that increased potassium intake is linked with a lower risk of stroke. More studies are needed to confirm these findings and to determine the benefits and risks of potassium supplements.

Cautions: Don't take potassium supplements unless your doctor recommends them. Too much, or too little, potassium can lead to serious health effects. Blood levels should be routinely monitored.

Side effects: Side effects can include nausea, vomiting, upset stomach, diarrhea and gas. Confusion and irregular heartbeat are less common.

Selenium

Recommended Dietary Allowance (RDA) for Adults

Life stage	Men and women	Pregnant	Breast-feeding
Age 19 or older	55 mcg/day		
Other		60 mcg/day	70 mcg/day

mcg = micrograms

Maximum daily intake (from all sources) unlikely to pose risk of side effects for adults: 400 mcg/day

Food sources include: Milk, broccoli, cabbage, poultry, fish, seafood, organ meats and whole-grain products. One slice of whole-wheat bread contains 10 mcg of selenium.

What it does: Selenium is a mineral associated with fat metabolism. It also has antioxidant properties, helping to prevent cell damage by neutralizing "free radicals" — molecules believed to be associated with aging and certain diseases.

What the research says: Some studies suggest that selenium may help prevent cancer and, possibly, heart disease. One small study found that those taking 200 mcg of selenium a day had lower rates of prostate, colon and total cancers than those taking a placebo. Another small study confirmed the prostate cancer finding. In 2001, a large study was launched to determine if selenium and vitamin E can help protect against prostate cancer, but results will take several years. However, at this time, the National Academy of Sciences does not recommend taking selenium in doses greater than the Daily Value (DV) of 70 mcg a day.

Cautions: See your doctor before taking selenium in doses above the DV of 70 mcg a day. If you're pregnant or breast-feeding, avoid selenium intake greater than the RDA (60 mcg daily if pregnant and 70 mcg daily if breast-feeding).

Side effects: Taking excessive amounts of selenium may cause hair and nail loss. Other symptoms may include gastrointestinal disturbance, skin rash, fatigue, irritability, tooth decay and nervous system abnormalities.

Zinc

Recommended Dietary Allowance (RDA) for Adults

Life stage	Men	Women	Pregnant	Breast-feeding
Age 19 or older	11 mg/day	8 mg/day		
Other			11 mg/day	12 mg/day

mg = milligrams

Maximum daily intake (from all sources) unlikely to pose risk of side effects for adults: 40 mg/day

Food sources include: Meat, fish, poultry, liver, eggs, milk, oysters, wheat germ and whole-grain products. A portion (3 ounces) of lean sirloin contains 5 mg of zinc.

What it does: Zinc is a mineral involved in wound healing, sense of taste and smell, growth and sexual maturation and is contained in enzymes that regulate metabolism.

What the research says: A 1996 study indicated that dissolving one particular formulation of a zinc lozenge in your mouth might reduce the duration and severity of cold symptoms. Some studies indicate that taking a daily multivitamin-mineral supplement containing zinc may increase immune response in older people, but other studies have shown that zinc may weaken the immune status of older people. Until more is known, it's better not to exceed the Daily Value (DV) of 15 mg, although vegetarians may need more than the RDAs shown in the chart. If you take zinc lozenges for a cold, stop taking them once your cold is gone. In addition, a 2001 study indicates that supplementation with zinc and certain antioxidants may slow the progression of age-related macular degeneration, but a small percentage of participants had side effects, so a doctor's supervision is important to determine proper doses.

Cautions: Don't take zinc if you have stomach or duodenal ulcers. See your doctor before taking zinc in doses above the DV of 15 mg or if you're taking a calcium supplement or tetracycline drugs. Zinc may interfere with absorption of these medicines. If applicable, don't take zinc in doses greater than the RDA for pregnant or breast-feeding women.

Side effects: Long-term, high doses of zinc (50 to 100 mg/day) can lower high-density lipoprotein (HDL) cholesterol (the "good" cholesterol), suppress immune system function, and interfere with the absorption of copper, which may result in microcytic anemia. Other side effects may include diarrhea, heartburn, nausea, vomiting and abdominal pain.

The final word: Food vs. supplements

If you want to improve your nutritional health, look first to a nutritionally balanced diet. The Mayo Clinic Healthy Weight Pyramid is your guide to good nutrition and a healthy weight. It emphasizes lower calorie foods that help you feel full.

The pyramid illustrates the types and amounts of foods you need to eat every day from five key food groups: vegetables, fruits, carbohydrates, protein/dairy and fats. Its triangular shape shows you where to focus when selecting foods. The most important foods — fruits and vegetables — form the foundation.

The bottom line? In most cases, you're far more likely to improve and protect your health by eating well than by taking supplements.

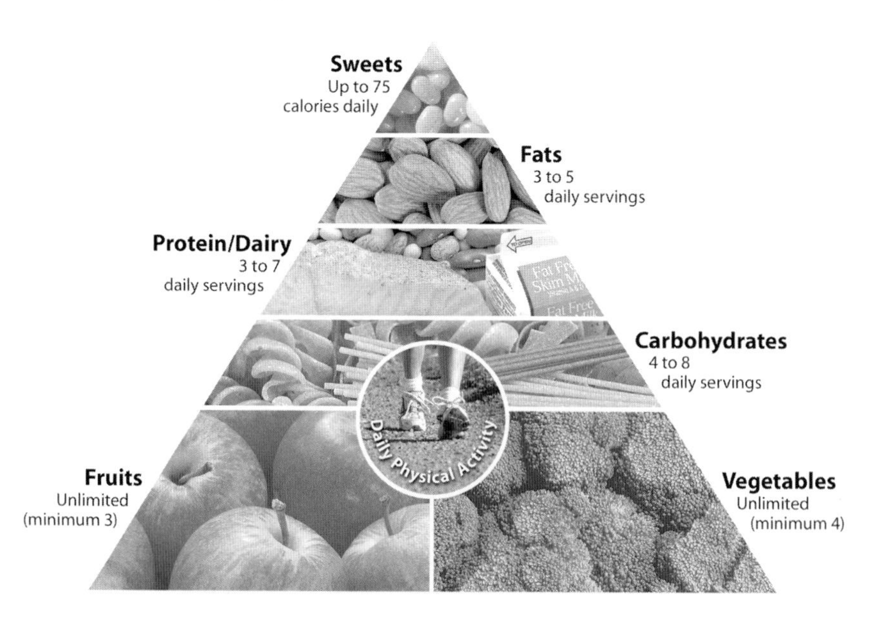

Mayo Clinic Healthy Weight Pyramid

Glossary

Atherosclerosis: Narrowing of the arteries due to the accumulation of cholesterol-containing fatty deposits. This can put you at risk for heart attack or stroke.

Carotenoids: Natural food pigments, usually yellow to red, widely found in plants and animals.

Electrolytes: Sodium, potassium and chloride are three minerals called electrolytes. They are important in regulating the water and chemical balance in your body.

Homocysteine: An amino acid that builds and maintains tissues. Elevated levels may increase your risk of heart attack, stroke or loss of circulation in your hands and feet.

Macular degeneration: A condition that occurs when tissue in the macula, the part of your retina responsible for central vision, deteriorates. It is the leading cause of severe vision loss in people age 50 and older.

Micronutrients: Vitamins and minerals are called micronutrients. Your body cannot make most of them, so you must get them from the foods you eat or from supplements.

Sarcoidosis: A disease, possibly related to the immune system, that can cause inflammation in many areas of the body. In most cases it affects the lungs.

Spina bifida: A birth defect affecting the spinal column. Consuming adequate quantities of vitamin B-9 during pregnancy may help prevent it. This vitamin is found naturally in some foods as folate, and in supplements and fortified foods in the form of folic acid.

Index

Daily values (DVs), 10-11

Enriched foods, 5

Fortified foods, 5

Healthy weight pyramid, 32

Interactions, 14

Multivitamins, 12-13

Premenstrual syndrome (PMS), 16-17

Recommended dietary allowances (RDAs), 10

Sunlight, 19-20

Whole foods, 6-7